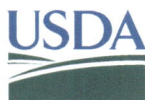

United States Department of Agriculture

I0467363

Economic Research Service

www.ers.usda.gov

Visit our website for more information on this topic:

www.ers.usda.gov/topics/food-safety/foodborne-illness.aspx

Access this report online:

www.ers.usda.gov/publications/eib-economic-information-bulletin/eib118.aspx

Download the charts contained in this report:

- Go to the report's index page www.ers.usda.gov/publications/ eib-economic-information-bulletin/eib118.aspx
- Click on the bulleted item "Download EIB118.zip"
- Open the chart you want, then save it to your computer

Recommended citation format for this publication:

Hoffmann, Sandra and Tobenna D. Anekwe. *Making Sense of Recent Cost-of- Foodborne-Illness Estimates,* EIB-118, U.S. Department of Agriculture, Economic Research Service, September 2013.

Cover photo credit: Shutterstock.

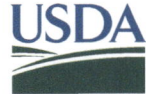

United States Department of Agriculture

Economic Research Service

Economic Information Bulletin Number 118

September 2013

Making Sense of Recent Cost-of-Foodborne-Illness Estimates

Sandra Hoffmann, shoffmann@ers.usda.gov

Tobenna D. Anekwe, tanekwe@ers.usda.gov

Abstract

Quantitative estimates of the economic and public health burden of foodborne illness, as well as the valuation of expected health benefits, are useful for evaluating the merit of food-safety regulations and assessing their effectiveness. Recent estimates of the cost of foodborne illnesses, based on U.S. Centers for Disease Control and Prevention (CDC) foodborne-disease figures, range widely. This variation could create confusion about the total cost burden of foodborne illnesses, as well as how different foodborne illnesses rank in terms of the health burdens they impose. Comparing these recent cost-of-foodborne-illness estimates, we find that the two primary drivers of differences in these estimates are differences in the number of diseases each study evaluates and the valuation methods used. Differences in relative pathogen rankings were due more to the number of diseases included in the analysis than to the method used to value the impact of the illnesses.

Keywords: Foodborne illness, health valuation, cost of illness, quality-adjusted life year, QALY, willingness to pay, value of a statistical life, VSL, EuroQol 5-Domain, EQ-5D, burden of disease, chronic sequelae, *Campylobacter, E. coli, Listeria,* norovirus, *Salmonella, Toxoplasma, Vibrio, Yersinia*

Acknowledgments

The authors want to thank Lisa Robinson, Harvard University; Alan Krupnick, Resources for the Future; Michael Batz, University of Florida; Robert Scharff, Ohio State University; and Juliana Ruzante, The Pew Charitable Trusts for their reviews of this report. Thanks also to ERS editor Priscilla Smith and ERS designer Wynnice Pointer-Napper.

Contents

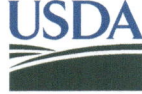

United States Department of Agriculture

A report summary from the Economic Research Service

September 2013

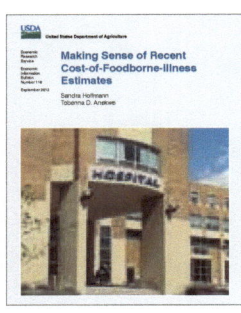

Find the full report
at *www.ers.usda.
gov/publications/eib-
economic-information-
bulletin/eib-118.aspx*

Making Sense of Recent Cost-of-Foodborne-Illness Estimates

Sandra Hoffmann and Tobenna D. Anekwe

What Is the Issue?

Estimates of the cost of foodborne illness play an important role in guiding Federal efforts to prevent foodborne illness in the United States. In 2000, the U.S. Department of Agriculture's Economic Research Service (ERS) estimated that the cost of illness from five major foodborne pathogens was $6.9 billion per year. In 2010 and 2012, new comprehensive cost-of-illness estimates were published for the first time in a decade. Scharff (2010; 2012) estimated the cost of foodborne illness in the United States to be as high as $152 billion, while Hoffmann et al. (2012) estimated that illness from 14 major pathogens in the United States cost $14.1 billion. The difference between these recent estimates could lead to confusion about the total economic burden of foodborne illnesses. This report examines these cost-of-illness estimates with a focus on analyzing the factors that drive differences between them. In this report, "cost of illness" is defined as the sum of treatment costs, the value of time lost to illness, and willingness to pay to prevent death. The studies we discuss estimated cost of illness in slightly different ways.

What Did the Study Find?

The apparently large differences between these cost-of-foodborne-illness estimates are due to basic choices in study design.

- The difference between Scharff's two estimates for the cost of all foodborne illness in the United States—$152 billion (2010) and $77.7 billion (2012)—is due primarily to changes in disease-incidence estimates from the Centers for Disease Control and Prevention (CDC). Estimation of the incidence of foodborne disease is a relatively new and rapidly evolving area of research. CDC notes that there is considerable uncertainty around its incidence estimates and advises that the difference between its 1999 and 2011 estimates not be viewed simply as a change in incidence.

- The difference between Scharff's 2012 estimates and Hoffmann et al.'s (2012) estimates is primarily driven by two factors.

  - **Number of pathogens included.** Scharff (2012) included estimates for foodborne illnesses caused by 30 of 31 identifiable pathogens plus foodborne illnesses for which no pathogen source can be identified in CDC's recent foodborne-disease-incidence estimates. By contrast, Hoffmann et al. (2012) included estimates for foodborne illness caused by only 14 identifiable pathogens that account for over 95 percent of

ERS is a primary source
of economic research and
analysis from the U.S.
Department of Agriculture,
providing timely informa-
tion on economic and policy
issues related to agriculture,
food, the environment,and
rural America.

the illnesses, hospitalizations, and deaths caused by all 31 identifiable pathogens (Scharff dropped 1 pathogen from his studies, thus the 30 for Scharff versus 31 for Hoffmann).

- **Valuation method.** Scharff's estimate of $152 billion included monetized quality-adjusted life years (QALYs) to account for pain and suffering caused by foodborne illness as well as the illnesses' impact on daily activities, such as employment. Hoffmann et al. (2012) did not use monetized QALYs. Instead, they used a cost-of-illness estimate for nonfatal outcomes and a willingness-to-pay (for reducing deaths) measure for fatal outcomes. Scharff also produced estimates that do not include monetized QALYs and are methodologically more comparable to Hoffmann et al. (2012). Two National Academy of Sciences committees and the U.S. Environmental Protection Agency's Scientific Advisory Board have found that current approaches to monetizing QALY loss are not reliable economic measures and advised against this practice. Cost of illness is an established practice recognized to be a reliable, though conservative, economic estimate of the burden of nonfatal illness.

Once these differences in study design are controlled for, the difference between Hoffmann et al. (2012) and Scharff (2012) is considerably smaller: $14.1 billion compared to $16.3 billion, respectively.

Methodological differences between Scharff (2012) and Hoffmann et al. (2012) have little impact on how pathogens rank by cost. When monetized QALYs are not included and the same 14 pathogens are considered, there is little difference in pathogen ranking. *Salmonella* (nontyphoidal) and *Toxoplasma gondii* are the first and second most costly foodborne pathogens in the United States.

How Was the Study Conducted?

This analysis is a synthesis and comparison of two prior cost-of-foodborne-illness studies (Scharff, 2012; Hoffmann et al., 2012). It includes a brief discussion of how these two studies compare to prior research based on earlier CDC estimates of the incidence of foodborne illness. The analysis compares published results and recalculates the mean cost of illness for comparable sets of pathogens to allow for more direct comparison of aggregate estimates across studies. It examines the impact of differences in the number of pathogens included in the studies, underlying disease-incidence estimates, valuation methodology, and uncertainty around estimates of disease burden on relative rankings of pathogens.

The studies that are central to this report's research are:

- Hoffmann, Sandra, Michael Batz, and J. Glenn Morris Jr. 2012. "Annual Cost of Illness and Quality-Adjusted Life Year Losses in the United States Due to 14 Foodborne Pathogens," *Journal of Food Protection* 75(7): 1291-1302.

- Scharff, Robert. 2010. *Health-related Costs from Foodborne Illness in the United States*. Produce Safety Project, Georgetown University, Washington, DC.

- Scharff, Robert. 2012. "Economic Burden from Health Losses Due to Foodborne Illness in the United States," *Journal of Food Protection* 75(1): 123-31.

Making Sense of Recent Cost-of-Foodborne-Illness Estimates

Sandra Hoffmann and Tobenna D. Anekwe

Introduction

Estimates of the economic cost of foodborne illness play an important role in guiding food safety policy. USDA, Economic Research Service (ERS) economists developed some of the first estimates of the cost of foodborne illnesses in the United States (Buzby et al., 1996; Crutchfield and Roberts, 2000). In 2000, ERS researchers estimated that five major foodborne pathogens caused illnesses that imposed a cost of $6.9 billion per year (Crutchfield and Roberts, 2000).[1] Since then, the literature on cost of foodborne illness has continued to grow. In 2010, Robert Scharff, professor of consumer sciences at Ohio State University, estimated a cost of $152 billion for *all* foodborne illnesses in the United States.

The above estimates are all based on 1999 CDC estimates of foodborne disease incidence (Mead et al., 1999). In 2011, CDC revised its estimates based on new research reflecting significant methodological changes in foodborne-disease-incidence estimation. Two 2012 studies estimated the cost of foodborne illness based on these new disease-incidence estimates (Scharff, 2012; Hoffmann et al., 2012). Cost estimates from these new studies range from $14.1 billion to $77.7 billion per year. The large difference in these totals has the potential to lead to confusion, particularly with regard to the total burden of foodborne illnesses in the United States.

This report provides an overview and comparison of these two new cost-of-foodborne-illness studies. We show that differences between these new estimates are primarily due to two factors: the number of pathogen-specific diseases whose impact is valued and the valuation methods employed. The source of the greatest difference between estimates is whether foodborne illnesses of unknown pathogen origin are included. Illnesses due to unknown pathogen origin are estimated to cause 80 percent of all foodborne illness. Such exposure also causes 56 percent of the hospitalizations, and 56 percent of deaths resulting from foodborne illness (Scallan et al., 2011b). The knowledge that most foodborne disease is due to these unspecified causes is critical to public health surveillance and to guiding epidemiological research priorities. It is not as useful in focusing food safety policy or management that can most effectively address problems for which the cause is understood. Scharff (2012) addresses the broad question of how large the total burden of U.S. foodborne illness is and includes illnesses of both known and unknown pathogen origin. Hoffmann and colleagues' estimates were part of a modeling effort designed to support regulatory policy and management decisionmaking and did not consider illnesses of unknown pathogen origin. The second greatest source of difference between the two sets of estimates is the valuation method used. Once these two factors are accounted for, most of the remaining difference between the two studies' estimates can be attributed to uncertainty inherent in the data underlying the estimates.

This report also examines the sensitivity of pathogen-specific cost-of-illness rankings to valuation method used and to the range of pathogens considered. We find that, when monetized quality-adjusted life year (QALY) estimates are not included and the same 14 pathogens are considered,

---

[1]Pathogens are bacteria, viruses, and parasites that cause illness.

there is little difference in how pathogens are ranked by cost of illness based on Scharff's (2012) and Hoffmann et al.'s (2012) estimates.

The context for these two studies is important for understanding why different methodological choices were made. This report begins with a discussion of the role of health-valuation estimates in Federal policy analysis. It next describes the major options for monetary and nonmonetary health-valuation metrics and discusses recent research developments that inform how such metrics should be used. It then looks at CDC foodborne-disease-incidence estimates and how they have changed since 1999. The report then turns to a comparison of the Scharff (2012) and Hoffmann et al. (2012) studies and explores how and why their estimates differ. Finally, the report examines the influence of methodological choices on relative rankings of foodborne pathogens by economic burden in the United States and identifies lessons regarding research needs.

Health-Valuation Methods and Their Use

Health-valuation estimates play two major roles in Federal policy analysis: (1) as a monetary measure of benefits used in cost-benefit analysis; and (2) as a nonmonetary measure of health impact used in cost-effectiveness analysis. Each type of analysis addresses different policy questions. Cost-benefit analysis (CBA) addresses the question of whether a program's expected aggregate benefits exceed its costs to society—i.e., is the program worth doing? As a result, both costs and benefits must be measured in monetary terms. Since the early 1980s, Federal agencies have been required to provide the U.S. Office of Management and Budget (OMB) with cost-benefit analyses of major proposed regulations prior to publishing proposed rules for public comment (U.S. Office of the President, 1993). These analyses help decisionmakers evaluate whether a new regulation is likely to increase the welfare of the American public. Cost-effectiveness analysis (CEA) addresses the question of how to allocate a limited budget as effectively as possible to achieve a defined goal, such as reducing foodborne illness—i.e., are we getting "the biggest bang for the buck"? Because benefits are not weighed against costs in CEA, benefits do not need to be measured in monetary terms. Instead, for programs protecting health, benefits are often measured using nonmonetary indices of the impact of illness on the quality of life. Since 2003, OMB has also required Federal agencies to include a CEA in regulatory impact analyses of major proposed rules when possible (U.S. OMB, 2003).

In recent years, the U.S. Food and Drug Administration (FDA) and the U.S. Department of Agriculture (USDA) also have begun to use pathogen-level health-valuation estimates to gain a clearer understanding of the relative public health burden of different foodborne hazards. Relative measures of health impacts can be critical for decisions about how to prioritize competing strategies for reducing disease risks. Risk-based prioritization is a cornerstone of the 2011 Food Safety Modernization Act (U.S. Congress, 2011).

Valuation measures are needed to compare the health burden of different foodborne pathogens. Most foodborne illness involves mild to moderate diarrhea that generally resolves without medical attention. But foodborne illness can lead to hospitalization—sometimes with serious conditions like sepsis or renal failure—and even death. Some foodborne illnesses also result in chronic conditions like arthritis, kidney disease, and chronic bowel inflammation. With such varied health outcomes, it is not possible to meaningfully compare the health impacts of different diseases using physical outcomes such as number of cases, hospitalizations, or deaths. Comparison of the public health impacts of diseases with such diverse outcomes requires use of either monetary or nonmonetary aggregate measures of the impact of illness.

Over the past two decades, both monetary and nonmonetary measures of the aggregate impact of health hazards have been developed and applied in Federal policy analysis. Federal agencies have historically used cost-of-illness estimates, sometimes augmented by estimates of willingness to pay to reduce risk of death, as a monetary measure. In more recent years, Federal agencies have begun to use nonmonetary, QALY metrics to compare the burden that different diseases place on society. Kuchler and Golan (1999), Viscusi (2008), and Robinson and Hammitt (2013) discuss the emergence of these practices in Federal agencies. Each of these aggregate measures has limitations.

Monetary Measures

In the basic economic theory underlying cost-benefit analysis, individuals are viewed as the best judge of their own welfare. Because individuals have limited budgets that they spend to meet a wide range of needs and desires, their willingness to pay for a good or service is used to measure how much they think expenditures on that good or service increase their welfare relative to other expenditures. An individual's willingness to pay to reduce the risk of becoming injured or ill reflects not only the individual's beliefs about all the ways the illness might affect things he or she cares about, but also the value the person places on other possible uses for scarce financial resources. Federal regulations such as food safety regulation, environmental regulation, and workplace safety regulation reduce the risk of an individual becoming ill or dying. As a result, standard economic theory views the correct measure of the benefits of these programs as the sum of the willingness of all individuals in society to pay for the reductions in risk of adverse health outcomes provided by the programs.

Many Federal public health or environmental policies result in small reductions in risk of death for a large number of people. A program that reduces the risk of death of individuals in a population of 1,000 by 1/1000 annually can be expected to prevent 1 premature death annually in this population, or save 1 "statistical life." The value of this reduced risk of mortality is expressed as the aggregate of individuals' willingness to pay for these small reductions in risk, a sum known as the value of a statistical life (VSL). A relatively large number of studies have estimated the VSL. Viscusi and Aldy (2003) and Lindhjem et al. (2011) provide recent reviews of this literature.

There has been far less empirical research on individuals' willingness to pay (WTP) to reduce the risk of nonfatal illness or injury (IoM, 2006; Andersson et al., 2011). In part, this is due to the fact that diseases vary greatly in symptoms, severity, and duration of impact on people's lives, while deaths are seen as less varied (Viscusi, 2008; Dickie and List, 2006). It is more difficult to justify spending for research on WTP to reduce risk of a particular illness because illness-speciific WTP can be used in a narrower set of analyses than studies of WTP to reduce risk of death. In addition, in past analyses, reductions in deaths have generally accounted for a very high percentage of the estimated value of benefits from environmental health and safety regulations that reduce risk of both illness and death (Dickie and List, 2006). As a result, for most diseases, estimates of individuals' WTP to reduce risk of illness are not available (IoM, 2006; Andersson et al., 2011; Robinson and Hammitt, 2013).

Where estimates of WTP to reduce risk of illness are not available, estimates of the financial impacts of illness are often used as a proxy. This is referred to as the "human capital" or "cost-of-illness" method of valuing health impacts. Typically, cost-of-illness estimates include the cost of treating illness as well as the opportunity cost of time lost to illness. Harrington and Portney published an article in 1987 that has become the standard reference on the theoretical relationship between willingness-to-pay and cost-of-illness measures of benefits from policies that reduce risk of illness. They show that willingness to pay to reduce risk of nonfatal illness can be broken down into the sum of four elements: medical expenses, the opportunity cost of time associated with illness, the disutility of experiencing the illness, and expenditures of money or time that individuals make to protect health.[2] In practice, cost-of-illness estimates generally include only medical expenses and estimates of the opportunity cost of time spent being ill and do not include estimates of disutility of illness or expenditures on self-protection. The opportunity cost of time associated with illness is also usually underestimated. Theoretically the opportunity cost of time should include the value of time that would have been spent at work, in leisure, and in household activities. It should include not only the time that the afflicted person spends being ill, but also the value of uncompensated time others spend caring for the ill person. Most cost-of-illness estimates, like ERS and Hoffmann et al. (2012) cost-of-foodborne-illness estimates, include only the lost wages of sick working people as the opportunity cost of time associated with illness.

---

[2]Disutility here refers to factors such as pain and discomfort, anxiety, depression, or a general dislike of being ill.

Scharff (2012) also includes the time parents spend caring for sick children valued at the average wage rate. Because cost-of-illness estimates usually do not include the disutility of illness or individuals' expenditures on reducing the health risk and typically underestimate the opportunity cost of time associated with illness, they are generally viewed as conservative, though practical, estimates of the value of reducing risk of nonfatal illness (Viscusi, 2008).

Nonmonetary Measures

Many public-health professionals have objected to monetary valuation of health based on the view that health is a "merit good," that is, a condition that cannot be traded off against other goods like education, defense, or future consumption. These experts also object to the fact that estimates of willingness to pay to reduce health risks reflect individuals' ability to pay and differences in preferences that arise from income inequality. As a result, public-health experts have advocated the use of nonmonetary measures of benefits to evaluate policies that protect health (Alder, 2006).

A group of nonmonetary measures known as quality-adjusted life year (QALY) measures were developed to assess the relative cost-effectiveness of alternative treatment or health care policy options and are widely used in countries with national health care programs (Zeckhauser and Shepard, 1976; Gold et al., 1996). These measures are now used by Federal agencies in CEA. Several QALY scales have been developed that integrate disease severity and duration for a wide range of health outcomes (see box, "The EuroQol 5-Domain and Measuring Quality-Adjusted-Life-Year Loss," p. 6). The quality of life associated with each outcome is rated on a scale of 0 to 1, where 1 is perfect health and 0 is death. Some QALY scales allow scores less than zero to permit the possibility that some conditions are viewed as worse than death. Robinson and Hammitt (2013) provide a brief introduction to QALYs, targeted to a policy audience. More comprehensive overviews include Gold et al. (1996), Gold et al. (2002), Institute of Medicine (IoM) (2006), and Lipscomb (2009).

In 2003, when OMB began asking agencies to provide CEA assessments of major regulations, many Federal agencies had little experience using QALY measures (IoM, 2006). A National Academy of Sciences (NAS) committee was convened at the request of several Federal agencies to provide recommendations on the use of QALY measures in Federal regulatory analysis. Among other guidance, the committee recommended use of QALY estimates based on population surveys rather than expert judgment because regulatory analysis needs to reflect public, not expert, preferences. The committee further recommended use of the EuroQol 5-Domain (EQ-5D) QALY scale because surveys of the U.S. population had been conducted to develop health-state severity ratings of 0 to 1 using the EQ-5D (IoM, 2006). The committee also recognized that other population-based ratings might be developed for the United States in the future.

Monetized Quality-Adjusted Life Years

A more controversial issue has been whether QALYs can be monetized and used in cost-benefit analysis to estimate the value of reducing health risks. The motivation for monetizing QALY loss is evident in the above discussion about the relationship between cost-of-illness and willingness-to-pay estimates. Few WTP estimates exist for many types of illness, and cost-of-illness estimates do not include the disutility associated with illness. Some aspects of the disutility of illness are captured by QALY metrics, like the EQ-5D (see box, p. 6). The argument for combining QALYs with cost of treatment is that doing so would move cost-of-illness estimates closer to full WTP.

The EuroQol 5-Domain and Measuring Quality-Adjusted-Life-Year Loss

The EuroQol 5-Domain (EQ-5D) is a standardized instrument used for describing and measuring impacts on health-related quality of life (EuroQol, 2013). The EQ-5D instrument uses five domains—mobility, ability for self-care, performance of usual activities, pain and discomfort, and anxiety and depression—to characterize health outcomes. Each domain can be rated on a scale of 1 to 3 (see table below). So, for example, the health outcome "moderate diarrhea" could be characterized as (1, 1, 2, 2, 1) on the five EQ-5D domains (i.e., no impact on mobility, self-care or anxiety/depression, and moderate impact on usual activities and pain/discomfort).

In nationally representative population surveys, respondents were asked to describe their current health using the EQ-5D instrument and then to rate their health on a scale of 0 to 1. These responses were then used to estimate health preference weights for each of 243 possible combinations of the 5 domains measured by the EQ-5D (Shaw, 2005).

In using the EQ-5D to value the impact of foodborne disease, detailed descriptions of the possible health outcomes of the disease, as well as their probability and duration, are developed. Different outcomes from specific foodborne illnesses (e.g., hospitalization for 5 days with sepsis due to a *Listeria* infection) are given a 5-digit domain characterization by researchers or a panel of experts using the EQ-5D instrument. Duration of the health outcome and preference weights, such as those estimated by Shaw et al. (2005) from a representative survey of the U.S. population, are then used to compute the quality-adjusted-life-year (QALY) loss associated with this particular disease outcome. For each pathogen, QALY loss for each health outcome caused by that pathogen is multiplied by the estimated number of people experiencing the outcome and then summed across outcomes caused by the pathogen to calculate pathogen-specific QALY loss.

EuroQol-5D quality-of-life-years scale domain, scores, and descriptions

Domain	Domain score		
	1	2	3
Mobility	I have no problems walking about	I have some problems walking about	I am confined to bed
Self-care	I have no problems with self-care	I have some problems washing or dressing myself	I am unable to wash or dress myself
Usual activities (e.g., work, housework, study, leisure)	I have no problems with performing my usual activities	I have some problems with performing my usual activities	I am unable to perform my usual activities
Pain/discomfort	I have no pain or discomfort	I have moderate pain or discomfort	I have extreme pain or discomfort
Anxiety/depression	I am not anxious or depressed	I am moderately anxious or depressed	I am extremely anxious or depressed

EuroQol-5D (EQ-5D) QALY scale = European quality of life quality-adjusted-life-years scale.

Source: Hoffmann, Sandra, Michael Batz, and J. Glenn Morris, Jr., 2012. "Annual Cost of Illness and QALY Losses in the United States Due To Fourteen Foodborne Pathogens," *Journal of Food Protection* 75(7): 1291-1302.

Serious questions have been raised in the economics literature about monetizing QALYs, mostly focused on how QALYs are currently monetized, but also on whether the scales used to elicit QALYs reflect preferences in a way that is consistent with economic measures (see appendix). Recently, two NAS committees and EPA's Scientific Advisory Board recommended that more research is needed to develop monetized QALYs that are consistent with the measures of welfare loss used in cost-benefit analysis and advised against monetizing QALYs based on current economics research (IoM, 2006; Cropper et al., 2007; National Research Council, 2008). See the appendix for a more indepth review of this literature.

Federal Agency Valuation Practice

Federal agencies vary in their approaches to monetary health valuation. USDA and EPA use willingness-to-pay estimates in valuing reductions in the risk of death resulting from their programs and generally use cost-of-illness estimates to value reductions in risk of morbidity (Viscusi, 2008). FDA uses willingness-to-pay estimates in valuing reductions in risk of death and a synthesis of cost-of-illness and monetized QALYs to value reductions in risk of illness (Viscusi, 2008). CDC uses cost-of-illness estimates to value illness and uses productivity loss to value mortality reductions (e.g., Grosse et al., 2007). A major reason for the differences in these agencies' practices is simply that agencies needed to make decisions about best practices at different points in time over the past 30 years, and research is constantly evolving (Viscusi, 2008). As is often the case, once practices are established, transition costs and a desire for consistency slow change. (For more extensive, accessible discussions of the history of health valuation in Federal cost-benefit analysis, see Robinson and Hammitt (2013) and Viscusi (2008).)

New Disease-Incidence Estimates

All analyses of the cost of foodborne illness build on estimates of the number of illnesses that occur in a typical year and their associated health outcomes. CDC is responsible for estimating foodborne-disease incidence for the U.S. population. CDC incidence estimates are based on all available data. This includes data from passive surveillance (i.e., voluntary reporting by health care providers and facilities), active surveillance by county and State public health authorities, outbreak investigations, and various population surveys (Scallan et al., 2011a; Scallan et al., 2011b). Yet, because of limitations in these data, CDC must also rely heavily on quantitative modeling involving researcher judgment to estimate the incidence of foodborne illness.

Estimation of the incidence of foodborne illness is a difficult task because people with foodborne illness do not always seek health care. Of those who do seek health care, only a small proportion of cases are reported to health departments, and only a small proportion of these reported cases are confirmed by laboratory testing, making it difficult to identify the pathogen that caused the illness. Determining whether food or another route of exposure caused the illness is also difficult because symptoms may not appear for days or weeks after exposure, and memory about everyday activities, like what one ate at different meals, is typically poor (U.S. FDA, 2012). As a result of all these factors, there is substantial underreporting of foodborne illness and significant uncertainty involved in distinguishing food from other sources of gastrointestinal illness.

For their most recent estimates, CDC researchers determined that data adequate for preparing national pathogen-specific incidence estimates were available for only 31 pathogens (Scallan et al., 2011a). CDC refers to these as "known" pathogens. For six of these pathogens, no routine surveillance data are collected. For the 25 pathogens that had surveillance data, CDC multiplied the number of illnesses by pathogen-specific multipliers to correct for underreporting, underdiagnosis, percentage of illness acquired domestically, and percentage of illness caused by foodborne exposure. There is uncertainty about the value of each of these multipliers. One advance that Scallan et al. (2011a; 2011b) made over Mead et al.'s (1999) earlier estimates was to provide estimates of uncertainty along with their mean estimates.

To provide an assessment of the overall burden of foodborne illness, Scallan et al. (2011b) also estimated the number of cases of foodborne illness in the United States for which no specific pathogen can be identified. They refer to this as illnesses caused by "unknown" foodborne pathogens. To estimate figures for disease caused by these pathogens, they estimated the total number of acute gastrointestinal illnesses using U.S. population survey data, then subtracted the number of illnesses caused by known pathogens. Multipliers were used to account for the proportion of acute gastrointestinal illnesses that is foodborne and the proportion that is acquired domestically, rather than through travel to foreign countries.

The degree of uncertainty in estimates of foodborne-disease incidence can be seen both in the size of the uncertainty bounds around Scallan et al.'s estimates and by comparing CDC's new estimates by Scallan et al. (2011a; 2011b) to earlier CDC work by Mead and coauthors (1999) (table 1). In an essay providing perspective on the 2011 incidence estimates, the editor of *Emerging Infectious Diseases*, which published Scallan et al.'s 2011 paper, explains that methodological differences play a significant role in the apparent difference between the Mead et al. (1999) and Scallan et al. (2011a, 2011b) disease-incidence estimates (Morris, 2011). The difference between Scallan et al.'s and Mead et al.'s estimates should not be interpreted as the change in foodborne-disease incidence between 1999 and 2011 (Scallan et al. 2011a, 2011b).

Making Sense of Recent Cost-of-Foodborne-Illness Estimates, EIB-118
Economic Research Service/USDA

Numerically, the two sets of estimates differ markedly. Mead et al. estimated that annually there were 76 million illnesses, 325,000 hospitalizations, and 5,000 deaths caused by eating contaminated food in the United States. Scallan et al. (2011a; 2011b) estimate that there are approximately 48 million illnesses, 128,000 hospitalizations, and 3,000 food-related deaths in the United States annually. These differences not only reflect changes in actual disease incidence over time, but also improvements in estimation methods and expansion of the set of pathogens evaluated. Scallan et al. estimate a 90-percent credible interval of 29 million to 71 million cases around their central estimate of 48 million cases (see table 1). Much of the difference between Scharff's 2010 estimate of $152 billion and his 2012 estimate of $77.7 billion is due to changes in CDC's incidence estimates.

Table 1

CDC estimates of annual incidence of foodborne illnesses acquired in the United States

Estimate	Number of pathogens	Cases	Hospitalizations	Deaths
		Million		
1999 estimates[a]	27 + unknown	76	325,000	5,000
		[not provided]	[not provided]	[not provided]
2011 estimates (total)	31 + unknown	47.8	127,839	3,037
		[28.7-71.1]	[62,529-215,562]	[1,492-4,983]
Major pathogens[b]	31	9.4	55,961	1,351
		[6.6 – 12.7]	[39,534 - 75,741]	[712-2,268]
Unspecified agents[c]	Unknown	38.4	71,878	1,686
		[19.8 -61.2]	[9,924-157,340]	[369-3,338]

Note: Brackets [ ] indicate a 90-percent credible interval. CDC = Centers for Disease Control and Prevention.
Sources: a = Mead et al., 1999; b = Scallan et al., 2011a; c = Scallan et al., 2011b.

Making Sense of Recent Cost-of-Foodborne-Illness Estimates, EIB-118
Economic Research Service/USDA

New Cost-of-Foodborne-Illness Estimates

The above discussion is central to understanding differences between recent cost-of-foodborne-illness estimates by Hoffmann et al. (2012) and Scharff (2012). In this section, we broadly describe the estimates from these studies. Table 2 provides a side-by-side comparison of the modeling approaches taken in these two studies. While there is an established practice in the United States of referring to estimates of the value of preventing foodborne illnesses as cost-of-foodborne-illness estimates, as described below, they generally combine cost-of-illness estimates for nonfatal illnesses with a willingness-to-pay-based estimate of the value of preventing premature deaths.

Hoffmann et al.'s (2012) estimates were developed as part of a risk-ranking model designed to improve information available for use in prioritization in food safety policy and management. They therefore focused on 14 pathogens that cause over 95 percent of the annual illnesses and hospitalizations and almost 98 percent of the deaths for which CDC can identify a pathogen cause (Scallan et al., 2011a). These pathogens include the 11 pathogens covered by FoodNet surveillance plus *Toxoplasma gondii, Clostridium perfringens*, and norovirus.[3] These three non-FoodNet pathogens are either leading causes of cases of foodborne illness or death from foodborne illness (Scallan et al., 2011a).

Hoffmann et al. accounted for acute outcomes (nonhospitalized illness, hospitalizations, and deaths) for all 14 pathogens and for chronic complications from *Campylobacter* (Guillain-Barré syndrome), *Cryptosporidium parvum* (recurring diarrhea), *E. coli* O157:H7 (hemolytic uremic syndrome [HUS], end-stage renal disease [ESRD]), STEC non-O157 (HUS and ESRD), a newly identified form of toxin-producing *E. coli*, and *Listeria* (chronic impairments in newborns). They estimated the cost of illness for these conditions using the lost wages of employed adults to measure the opportunity cost of time imposed by the illnesses. They included the cost of outpatient visits, emergency room visits, and hospitalization. They included the cost of medications administered in the hospital, but not those taken by outpatients because outpatient medications represent a tiny percentage of total cost of medical treatment. For example, for *E. coli* O157:H7, ERS cost-of-foodborne-illness estimates show that medicines used to treat outpatient cases accounted for less than a tenth of a percent of the pathogen's total cost of illness (USDA, ERS Foodborne Illness Cost Calculator, accessed April 2012). Hoffmann et al. (2012) value deaths using a VSL estimate of $7.9 million ($ 2009) updated from a 1997 meta-analysis by EPA by adjusting for both inflation and real income growth (EPA, 2010a). In total, Hoffmann et al. (2012) estimated that the mean annual cost of foodborne illness from the 14 pathogens in their study is $14.1 billion.

Scharff's (2012) goal was to provide an estimate of the total burden of foodborne disease in the United States. As a result, he included all foodborne illnesses, whether or not a pathogen cause could be identified. Scharff included chronic arthritis resulting from *Campylobacter, Salmonella, Shigella*, and *Yersinia* infections in addition to the chronic conditions included in the ERS (2000) estimates.

Scharff's most-cited estimate of $77.7 billion uses cost of treatment plus monetized QALYs to estimate the value of preventing these illnesses. He calls this an "enhanced" cost-of-illness estimate.

---

[3]FoodNet is an active disease surveillance system involving the collaboration of 10 State departments of public health, CDC, USDA's Food Safety and Inspection Service, and FDA. FoodNet was established in 1995 and tracks laboratory-confirmed cases of illness caused by *Campylobacter, Cryptosporidium, Cyclospora, Listeria, Salmonella,* Shiga toxin-producing *Escherichia coli* (STEC) O157 and non-O157, *Shigella, Vibrio*, and *Yersinia.*

Table 2

Side-by-side comparison of components included in estimates by Hoffmann et al. (2012) and Scharff (2012)

	Scharff enhanced	Scharff basic	Hoffmann et al.
Number of pathogens studied	30	30	14
Accounted for acute illness	✓	✓	✓
Accounted for the following chronic outcomes:			
Guillain-Barré syndrome due to *Campylobacter*	✓	✓	✓
Chronic impairments in newborns due to *Listeria*	✓	✓	✓
HUS & ESRD due to *E. coli* O157:H7	✓	✓	✓
Recurring diarrhea due to *C. parvum*	-------	-------	✓
HUS & ESRD due to STEC non-O157	-------	-------	✓
Chronic arthritis due to *Campylobacter*, *Salmonella*, *Shigella*, and *Yersinia*	✓	✓	-------
VSL used to value premature deaths	$7.3 million	$7.3 million	$7.9 million
	——— $ 2010 ———		*$ 2009*
Estimate includes monetized QALYs?	✓	-------	-------
Included outpatient over-the-counter and prescription drugs?	✓	✓	-------

HUS = hemolytic uremic syndrome. ESRD = end-stage renal disease. STEC = shiga toxin-producing *Escherichia coli*. QALYs = quality-adjusted life years. VSL = value of a statistical life.
Source: USDA, Economic Research Service analysis.

This estimate uses monetized QALY loss net of lost wages of ill employed adults to value disutility *and* productivity loss due to illness. A constant value of a statistical life year (VSLY) is used to monetize QALY loss from morbidity caused by acute foodborne illness (see appendix).

Scharff (2012) also includes an estimate of $51 billion that uses cost of treatment plus productivity loss to value nonfatal illnesses and a VSL estimate of $7.3 million ($ 2010) to value the reduction of mortality risk. He refers to this as a "basic" cost-of-illness estimate. This estimate is more analogous to Hoffmann et al.'s (2012) estimate than the enhanced estimate because neither Scharff's basic estimate nor Hoffmann et al.'s estimate use monetized QALYs. Unlike Hoffmann et al. (2012), though, Scharff includes lost wages for parents of sick children as well as for employed victims of illness in his basic estimates. Scharff (2012)'s estimates are based on CDC's 2011 disease incidence estimates (Scallan et al., 2011a; Scallan et al., 2011b). Like ERS (2000), Scharff includes prescribed and over-the-counter drugs used to treat nonhospitalized cases of illness. Scharff uses Viscusi and Aldy's (2003) mean VSL estimate of $6.7 million ($ 2000), updated to 2010 for changes in inflation and real income.

Explaining the Differences Between New Cost-of-Foodborne-Illness Estimates

To understand why these cost-of-illness estimates differ so greatly, it is necessary to understand the scope of the analysis behind each estimate and the valuation methods used. Once both of these factors are accounted for, remaining differences in overall disease-burden estimates fall well within the range implied by CDC's disease-incidence uncertainty bounds. That is, the number of pathogens evaluated, differences in valuation methods, and uncertainty about disease incidence can fully account for differences in recent aggregate estimates that, at first reading, seem so significant.

Diseases Considered

Much of the difference between cost-of-illness estimates is due to the number of illnesses included in each study. CDC estimates there are 9.4 million cases of foodborne illness each year in the United States for which pathogen causes can be identified and 38.4 million additional cases for which the pathogen cause cannot be identified (see table 1). Illnesses from known pathogens are estimated to result in disproportionately more serious outcomes than illnesses attributed to unknown pathogens. CDC estimates indicate that known pathogens are twice as likely to cause a hospitalization as unknown pathogens are and over three times as likely to cause a death.

As noted above, Scharff includes these unknown pathogens and Hoffmann and colleagues do not. Unknown pathogens account for two-thirds of Scharff's (2012) basic cost-of-illness estimates ($34.2 million) and a little under 60 percent of cost of illness when monetized QALY loss ($45.2 million) is used to capture lost productivity and disutility (table 3).[4] Ninety-six percent of the cost of illness that Scharff estimates is caused by known pathogens is due to the same 14 pathogens included in Hoffmann et al. (2012) ($16.3 billion compared to $16.9 billion per year using Scharff's basic estimate).

Methods Used To Value Health Impacts

Judgments about valuation method are also important to understanding the differences in the estimates. Both decisions about whether to use monetized QALYs and decisions about how to conduct conventional cost-of-illness analysis affect the relative size of the two sets of estimates.

The difference between Scharff's (2012) basic estimate of $51 billion and enhanced estimate of $77.7 billion (see table 3) reflects differences in how disutility of illness and time lost to illness are treated. Scharff's basic estimate includes lost wages of the sick person and uses lost wages to value the time of parents who are caring for sick children, but it does not include a measure of disutility of illness. Scharff's enhanced estimate uses monetized QALYs to measure lost wages of the sick person and the disutility of illness but also includes use of wages to value the time parents spend caring for sick children. Comparing the two Scharff estimates, monetization of QALYs adds roughly 50 percent to his conventional cost-of-illness estimates.

---

[4]Scharff (2012) does not value the impact of *Mycobacterium bovis*, which is included in the 31 pathogens for which CDC can estimate foodborne-disease incidence.

Table 3

Comparison of cost-of-foodborne-illness estimates by ERS, Scharff, and Hoffmann et al.

Valuation method	CDC incidence estimate used	Number of pathogens included	Cost of foodborne illnesses ($ billion per year)			
			ERS (2000)	Scharff (2010)	Scharff (2012)	Hoffmann et al. (2012)
			$ 2000	*$ 2009*	*$ 2010*	*$ 2009*
Cost of illness	Mead et al. (1999)	5	$6.9			
	Scallan et al. (2011)	30 known + all unknown			$51.0	
	Scallan et al. (2011)	30 known			$16.9	
	Scallan et al. (2011)	14 known from Hoffmann et al.			$16.3	$14.1
Cost of illness + monetized QALYs	Mead et al. (1999)	27 known + all unknown		$152		
	Scallan et al. (2011)	30 known + all unknown			$77.7	
	Scallan et al. (2011)	30 known			$32.5	

QALYs = quality-adjusted life years. CDC = Centers for Disease Control and Prevention
Source: USDA, Economic Research Service analysis.

A Note on Chronic Sequelae

Both Hoffmann et al. (2012) and Scharff (2012) expand on the set of long-term health impacts included in past ERS estimates (Buzby and Roberts, 1996; Crutchfield and Roberts, 2000). Hoffmann et al. (2012) also include recurring diarrhea from *Cryptosporidium parvum* and QALY estimates only for the contribution of *Toxoplasma* infections to vision loss and congenital impacts. Scharff does not. Scharff expands on the ERS estimates by adding the impact of reactive arthritis resulting from infections with *Campylobacter, Salmonella, Shigella,* and *Yersinia*; Hoffmann et al. do not. Because Scharff does not report separate estimates for chronic impacts, it is not possible to tell how this difference in the chronic impacts considered contributes to differences in total cost-of-illness estimates in the two studies.

In most estimates of the health benefits from policies that reduce risk of both illness and death, reductions in deaths account for most of the estimated benefits (Dickie and List, 2006). The results in these estimates show that chronic illness is also important. Chronic impacts accounted for 16 percent of morbidity costs in Hoffmann et al. (2012). Hoffmann et al. (2012) estimated nonmonetized QALY loss for the 14 illnesses included in their study. Seventy-three percent of this QALY loss was due to death following acute illnesses, and 20 percent was due to chronic illness. Only 7 percent of the QALY loss was due to nonhospitalized and hospitalized acute illness that did not result in death.

Evidence from both studies suggests that chronic impacts are more important in QALY estimates than in cost-of-illness estimates. Sharff finds chronic illness to be significant in explaining his enhanced, but not his basic, estimates. Hoffmann et al. find that Guillain-Barré syndrome accounts for 56 percent of the cost of illness from *Campylobacter*, but 77 percent of the QALY loss. While this does not explain the difference between Scharff's basic and Hoffmann et al.'s cost-of-illness estimates, it does show that both studies point to the contribution of chronic impacts on the burden of foodborne illness. The implications of this for future research are discussed toward the end of this report.

Interpreting Results in Light of Uncertainty

CDC estimates that there is a 90-percent likelihood that total incidence of foodborne illness in the United States could be anywhere between 28.7 million and 71.1 million cases annually (Scallan et al., 2011a; Scallan et al., 2011b). CDC also estimates uncertainty bounds for each pathogen. Scharff (2012) and Hoffmann et al. (2012) use CDC's pathogen-specific uncertainty modeling to evaluate uncertainty around their mean cost estimates for each pathogen.

Confidence intervals around Hoffmann et al.'s estimates tend to be smaller than those around Scharff's (fig. 1). For example, for *Campylobacter*, Scharff's mean basic estimate is $1,560 million ($ 2010) with a 90-percent confidence interval of $437 million to $4,031 million. Hoffmann et al. estimate a mean annual cost of illness for *Campylobacter* of $1,747 million ($ 2009) with a 90-percent confidence interval of $841 million to $4,151 million. But at a practical level, it is important to see that for individual pathogens, Hoffmann et al.'s mean estimate and Scharff's mean basic estimate consistently fall within each other's uncertainty bounds (see figure 1).

It is also important to keep in mind that much of the uncertainty about the burden of foodborne illness is unquantified. CDC estimates that 80 percent of foodborne illnesses are caused by unspecified agents, where the pathogen and therefore the health outcomes (other than death) are mostly unknown.

In aggregate, Hoffmann et al. (2012) estimate that cost of illness for 14 major pathogens could range from as low as $4.35 billion to as high as $33.0 billion ($ 2009). Scharff (2012) estimates that the 90-percent credible interval around his mean basic estimate of $16.9 billion for 30 foodborne illnesses due to known causes is $8.4 billion to $29.2 billion ($ 2010). While it is not possible based on published information to estimate an uncertainty bound for Scharff's analysis around the 14 pathogens included in Hoffmann et al. (2012), Scharff's mean estimate of $16.3 billion/year for the 14 pathogens included in Hoffmann et al. (2012) falls in the middle of Hoffmann et al.'s range of $4.45 billion to $33.0 billion for these same pathogens. Hoffmann et al.'s total estimate of $14.1 billion/year also falls in the middle of Scharff's (2012) range for his basic estimate for the 30 known pathogens included in his study.

Figure 1

Annual cost of illness due to the five most expensive foodborne pathogens in the United States

$ billion

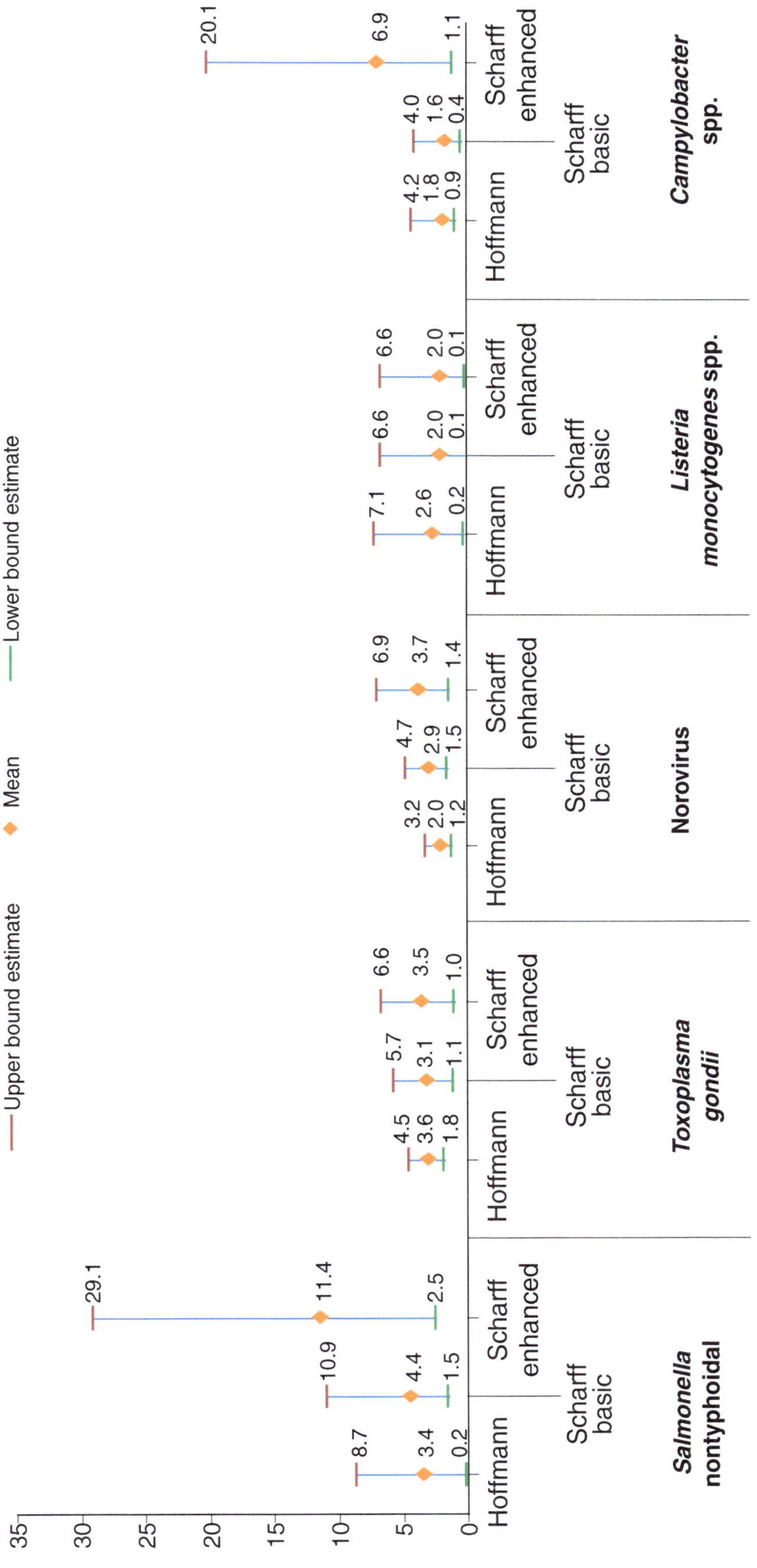

Legend: — Upper bound estimate   ◆ Mean   — Lower bound estimate

Source: USDA, Economic Research Service analysis.

Making Sense of Recent Cost-of-Foodborne-Illness Estimates, EIB-118
Economic Research Service/USDA

Impact on Pathogen Rankings

Relative rankings by public health burden are used to help inform priority setting for food safety efforts by government and industry. Table 3 shows how pathogens rank based on Hoffmann et al.'s (2012) estimates and Scharff's (2012) estimates. The table presents rankings for the 14 pathogens included in Hoffmann et al. (2012) as a means of assessing the influence of valuation methodology on rankings. It also presents rankings for the 30 pathogens in Scharff (2012) as a means of evaluating the influence that limiting the set of pathogens considered has on rankings.

When the set of pathogens considered is limited to the 14 included in Hoffmann et al., differences in rankings are primarily driven by whether monetized QALYs are included in the cost-of-illness estimates. Rankings of the 14 pathogens based on Scharff's basic estimate and based on Hoffmann et al.'s estimate do differ, but the rankings are also highly correlated (rank correlation coefficient of 0.96), indicating that the differences are not large. When the rankings are each split into the top 5, middle 5, and bottom 4 pathogens, both rankings agree on which pathogens fall into each group. Within these groupings, differences in rankings are slight. For example, norovirus (a highly contagious pathogen generally producing a fairly mild illness) ranks slightly higher in Scharff (2012) than in Hoffmann et al. (2012). This may reflect the fact that Scharff includes the cost of over-the-counter drugs, but Hoffmann et al. do not. Most of the mild cases do not result in even a doctor's visit. In contrast, *Vibrio vulnificus* (which results in very serious illness and a relatively high rate of death) ranks 7th in Hoffmann et al. and 9th in Scharff.

Differences in rankings are greater, but still not large, for these 14 pathogens when rankings of estimates that include monetized QALYs are compared to those that do not. The rank correlation of Scharff's enhanced estimates (which include monetized QALYs) with his basic estimates (which do not) is 0.73. The rank correlation of Scharff's enhanced estimates and Hoffmann et al.'s estimates is 0.69. Again, the same pathogens fall into each third of the rankings across methods, but there is more movement within each third. *Campylobacter* spp., which ranked 5th in both Hoffmann et al. and Scharff's basic estimates, ranks 2nd when monetized QALYs are used in the cost-of-illness estimates. This reflects the increased weight this method is placing on the chronic complications of illnesses caused by *Campylobacter*. One of the most striking comparisons is that the cost per case for *Shigella* in Scharff's estimate with monetized QALY loss is five times higher than his basic estimate, $9,551, compared to $1,956. The difference reflects the sensitivity of the monetized QALYs to arthritis that can result from *Shigella* infections. This results in its rise from 10th to 6th place ranking. In contrast, the cost per case of *E. coli* O157:H7, which moves down in ranking from 6th to 8th, is relatively unchanged: $9,606 in Scharff's basic estimate compared to $10,048 when monetized QALYs are included. *E. coli* O157:H7 has received a great deal of public attention because it can result in kidney disease and associated death, particularly in young children.

Including 30 known pathogens in the analysis rather than limiting it to 14 major pathogens affects which pathogens rank 10th to 15th; but the rankings of the top 9 pathogens are unaffected. Most notably, *Giardia intestinalis* and *Staphylococcus* move up into the top 15 pathogens. *Cyclospora cayetanensis*, which ranked 14th among the 14 pathogens in Hoffmann et al. (2012) for all estimation methods, moves down to 25th based on Scharff's basic estimate and 24th when he includes monetized QALYS.

From a disease-management perspective, though, the most important lesson is that *Campylobacter*, norovirus, *Listeria monocytogenes, Salmonella* nontyphoidal, and *Toxoplasma gondii* rank in the top five pathogens regardless of the valuation method or the number of pathogens included in the analysis. With the exception of *Vibrio vulnificus*, the same is true of the pathogens that rank 6th through 10th. Hoffmann et al. (2012) also estimate QALY loss, but do not monetize it. The same five pathogens rank in the top five on nonmonetized QALY loss. Four of the five pathogens that rank from 6th to 10th on cost of illness measures also do so for these nonmonetized QALY loss estimates.

Table 4

Pathogen ranking by cost of illness

| | Hoffmann et al. (2012) | | Scharff (2012) basic cost of illness | | | | Scharff (2012) enhanced cost of illness (cost of illness with monetized QALYs) | | | |
| | Cost of illness | | 14 pathogens included in Hoffmann et al. (2012) | | All 30 known pathogens | | 14 pathogens included in Hoffmann et al. (2012) | | All 30 known pathogens | |
Rank	Pathogen	$ millions ($ 2009)	Pathogen	$ millions ($ 2010)	Pathogen	$ millions ($ 2010)	Pathogen	$ millions ($ 2010)	Pathogen	$ millions ($ 2010)
1	Salmonella, nontyphoidal	3,309	Salmonella, nontyphoidal	4,430	Salmonella, nontyphoidal		Salmonella, nontyphoidal	11,391	Salmonella, nontyphoidal	
2	Toxoplasma gondii	2,973	Toxoplasma gondii	3,100	Toxoplasma gondii		Campylobacter spp.	6,879	Campylobacter spp.	
3	Listeria monocytogenes	2,577	Norovirus	2,896	Norovirus		Norovirus	3,677	Norovirus	
4	Norovirus	2,002	Listeria monocytogenes	2,025	Listeria monocytogenes		Toxoplasma gondii	3,456	Toxoplasma gondii	
5	Campylobacter spp.	1,747	Campylobacter spp.	1,560	Campylobacter spp.		Listeria monocytogenes	2,040	Listeria monocytogenes	
6	Clostridium perfringens	309	E. coli O157:H7	607	E. coli O157:H7		Shigella spp.	1,254	Shigella spp.	
7	Vibrio vulnificus	291	Yersinia enterocolitica	409	Yersinia enterocolitica		Yersinia enterocolitica	1,107	Yersinia enterocolitica	
8	E. coli O157:H7	255	Clostridium perfringens	382	Clostridium perfringens		E. coli O157:H7	635	E. coli O157:H7	
9	Yersinia enterocolitica	252	Vibrio vulnificus	268	Vibrio vulnificus		Clostridium perfringens	466	Clostridium perfringens	
10	Shigella spp.	121	Shigella spp.	257	Shigella spp.		Vibrio vulnificus	268	Giardia intestinalis	772
11	Vibrio spp. other	107	Vibrio spp. other	146	Giardia intestinalis	185	Vibrio spp. other	176	Vibrio vulnificus	268
12	Cryptosporidium parvum	47	Cryptosporidium parvum	118	Vibrio spp. other	146	Cryptosporidium parvum	168	Vibrio spp. other	176
13	STEC non-O157	24	STEC non-O157	101	Staphylococcus	130	STEC non-O157	154	Staphylococcus	168
14	Cyclospora cayetanensis	2	Cyclospora cayetanensis	11	Cryptosporidium spp.	118	Cyclospora cayetanensis	17	Cryptosporidium parvum	168
15					STEC non-O157	101			STEC non-O157	154

QALYs = quality-adjusted life years.
Source: USDA, Economic Research Service analysis.

Making Sense of Recent Cost-of-Foodborne-Illness Estimates, EIB-118
Economic Research Service/USDA

Research Needs

This analysis of Hoffmann et al. (2012) and Scharff (2012) suggests a number of research needs. It is clear from the differences in estimates provided that there is a need to learn from and to contribute to the continuing research on health-valuation methods. While use of a constant VSLY is not supported by current economic research, it is also not clear that valuing all reductions in risk of death using the same VSL accurately reflects individuals' WTP to reduce mortality risks. In addition, most VSL estimates are based on choices made in labor markets, and we do not know whether WTP to reduce risk of death from foodborne illness is different from this. There is a need to more fully capture the impacts of foodborne illness on people's time. Clearly, lost wages provide a very conservative estimate. Further work is also needed to assess the importance of including the disutility of illness in health-valuation estimates. If the disutility of illness is significant, then it will be important to know how it varies by illness.

Are there alternatives to using conservative cost-of-illness estimates or using QALYs monetized with a constant VSLY? Ideally, for CBA one would like to have estimates of WTP to reduce risk of the specific health outcomes of concern. Studies estimating WTP to reduce risk of illness do exist, although they are fewer in number than VSL studies. Most of the disease-specific WTP studies focus on reduction in risk of illness due to environmental exposures (e.g., health conditions such as asthma, bronchitis, or melanoma) that are not typically associated with foodborne illness (Vassanadumrongdee et al., 2004; Brouwer and Bateman, 2005, Hunt and Ferguson, 2010; Hammitt and Haninger, 2010). The range of health outcomes associated with foodborne illness caused by pathogens is relatively limited, centered mainly on diarrhea of varying duration and severity, renal disease, birth defects, stillbirths, arthritis, and chronic gastrointestinal disease. One possibility would be to invest in these studies. Two recent studies have looked at willingness to pay to reduce the risk of gastrointestinal illness from drinking contaminated water (Adamowicz et al., 2011; Viscusi et al., 2012). Hammitt and Haninger (2007) estimate WTP to reduce the risk of short-duration foodborne gastrointestinal illness.

An interesting alternative is emerging from stated-preference research that attempts to estimate WTP to reduce the risk of QALY loss using a variety of QALY indices (Gyrd-Hansen, 2003; Pinto-Prades et al., 2009; Hammitt and Haninger, 2011). In these studies, individuals are asked what they would forgo to avoid experiencing particular health states with specified durations. Because QALY health states may apply to multiple sets of illness, this has the potential to provide greater flexibility in estimating WTP to reduce the risk of a broader range of nonfatal health outcomes. Andersson, Sundström, and Hammitt (2011) compare WTP to reduce the risk of fatal and nonfatal illness and WTP per QALY in the context of efforts to reduce the risk of foodborne salmonellosis in Sweden. While this is still a relatively small literature, it is an encouraging development that may be capable of providing estimates of the monetary value of different health states as measured by QALYs.

If this last approach is pursued, thought must still be given to what is being measured by QALY indices and how this can be integrated into cost-benefit analysis. In all stated-preference research, such as these QALY valuation studies, the good being valued is explicitly defined. In these studies, the QALY index is used to define the health outcomes being valued. QALY indices were developed for use in clinical settings and in health policy settings that are often looking at healthcare. Researchers and analysts need to examine whether the attributes used to define QALYs in clinical settings are the same attributes that individuals would consider in making the choices implied by public policy decisions.

Hammitt and Haninger (2011) find that the name of the illness affects willingness to pay, particularly for milder diseases. This may be an example where risk attitudes like familiarity, controllability, or dread may affect WTP to reduce the risk of a disease (Slovic, 1987). But there may also be nonattitudinal factors related to certain illnesses that may affect WTP, such as how a particular disease affects a person's ability to care financially for family members.

Analysis looking solely at nonmonetized QALYs points to the importance of chronic illness to the public health burden of foodborne illness. As seen above in the *Campylobacter* estimates, where serious chronic impacts exist, they can account for most of the nonfatal impacts of illness. New research continues to enhance our understanding of the chronic impacts of infectious disease. For example, studies following victims of a major failure in the Walkerton, Canada, water treatment system suggest there may be significant links between infection with toxin-producing *E. coli* and hypertension (Garg et al. 2005). Because these chronic illnesses can have serious impacts on health over long periods of time, reducing the risk of these illnesses may be an important part of the benefit of reducing foodborne disease. As a result, continued attention by both epidemiologists and health economists to chronic impacts is needed.

The fact that we do not know the pathogen source of most of the foodborne illness in the United States limits our ability to understand how to control such illness. It is important to improve our understanding of the cause of these illnesses. Scharff's (2012) analysis of the welfare impacts of foodborne illness due to unknown pathogen origin can inform decisions about how much is worth spending on improving knowledge about the causes of these illnesses. Continuing research should also update valuation estimates as treatment and treatment costs change.

Conclusions

There is a large degree of agreement between recent cost-of-foodborne-illness estimates by Scharff (2012) and Hoffmann et al. (2012). While specific costs per pathogen vary between the two studies and the rank order of pathogens by cost also varies somewhat, many major conclusions about the economic burden of foodborne illness in the United States are consistent across the two studies. Nontyphoidal *Salmonella* and *Toxoplasma gondii* are the first and second most costly foodborne pathogens, respectively, in the United States in both studies. In both studies, the next three most costly foodborne pathogens are norovirus, *Listeria monocytogenes*, and *Campylobacter* spp., with slight variation in the order. To the extent that pathogen rankings are relevant to priority setting, the robustness of these findings should give decisionmakers confidence about which pathogens are causing the greatest public health burden.

Glossary

CBA   Cost-benefit analysis (CBA) is a systematic process for estimating the net benefits of a project in monetary terms. CBA is used in evaluating and designing major Federal regulations in the United States. Most other developed countries also require CBA to inform decisions about major government regulations.

CEA   Cost-effectiveness analysis (CEA) is a systematic process for comparing the relative costs of achieving comparable project outcomes. Project costs are calculated in monetary terms. Project benefits are expressed in nonmonetary terms. CEA is used to rank alternative strategies for achieving a goal. Since 2003, Federal agencies have been required to consider CEA in development of major regulations.

HRQL   The health-related quality of life (HRQL) is a scale that measures an individual's satisfaction with aspects of her or his life, usually those relevant to medical decisionmaking. Most HRQL scales measure the impact of disease and/or medical treatment on physical, social/role, psychological/emotional, and cognitive functioning. The EuroQol-5D (EQ-5D) is one HRQL scale (see box, "The EuroQol 5-Domain and Measuring Quality-Adjusted-Life-Year Loss," p. 6).

QALY   The quality-adjusted life year (QALY) is a nonmonetary measure of the burden of disease that reflects both the quality and duration of life and health conditions. Numerically, QALYs are calculated by multiplying the time spent in a health condition of interest by an HRQL score for that condition. This QALY estimate is then compared to the QALY value for expected remaining life spent in normal or perfect health to calculate QALY loss or gain. QALY estimates are widely used to assess the cost-effectiveness of health care policy and medical treatment options. Since 2003, U.S. Federal agencies have increasingly used them in CEA supporting analysis of major Federal regulations. QALYs are one measure in the family of health-adjusted life year (HALY) metrics that also include disability-adjusted life year (DALY) measures.

VSL   The value of a statistical life (VSL) is individuals' willingness to pay for small changes in their risk of death divided by the change in risk. If WTP for a 1 in 10,000 reduction in risk of death over the next year is $600, the VSL is $6,000,000. The use of the term a "statistical life" refers to the fact that while, for an individual, there is a reduction in risk of death over a specified time period, in aggregate across a population, this leads to an expected reduction in deaths over the time period.

VSLY   The value of a statistical life year (VSLY) is individuals' willingness to pay for a small reduction in risk of shortening their life expectancy by one year. In policy analysis, the VSLY is usually calculated as the average VSL for a population divided by average remaining life expectancy of that population discounted to present value. In a simplified example taken from Robinson and Hammitt (2013), if there were no discounting and the average age of a population in a study that estimates a VSL of $6 million is 40 and with an average life expectancy of 75, then the VSLY would be $6 million divided by 35 or $279,000. As discussed in the appendix, there is significant evidence that the VSLY varies by age and life expectancy.

WTP   Willingness to pay (WTP) is an individual's willingness to pay for a good or service. The term is used in this paper to refer to estimates of an individual's willingness to pay to reduce risk of either death or illness. In practice, WTP to protect health is measured either from market data or survey data. Examples of market data used to estimate WTP to protect health include wage rates that vary by job risk or the data on price and quantity of consumer products that vary in their safety risk. Stated-preference health-valuation surveys either ask respondents whether they would buy a specific product or service that reduces health risks by a specific amount at a stated price or asks respondents to choose among an array of such products or services that vary in characteristics including safety, risk, and price.

References

Adamowicz, Wiktor, Diane Dupont, Alan Krupnick, and Jing Zhang. 2011. "Valuation of Cancer and Microbial Disease Risk Reductions in Municipal Drinking Water: An Analysis of Risk Context Using Multiple Valuation Methods," *Journal of Environmental Economics and Management* (6): 213-26.

Alder, Matthew. 2006. "QALYs and Policy Evaluation: A New Perspective." *Yale Journal of Health Policy, Law and Ethics* (6): 1-581.

Aldy, Joseph, and W. Kip Viscusi. 2007. "Age Differences in the Value of Statistical Life: Revealed Preference Evidence," *Review of Environmental Economics and Policy*, 1(2): 241-60.

Andersson, Henrick, Kristian Sundström, and James Hammitt. 2011. "Willingness-to-pay and QALYs: What Can We Learn about Valuing Foodborne Risk?" Working Paper. Accessed April 2013 at: http://neeo.univ-tlse1.fr/3014/1/11.21.355.pdf

Bleichrodt, Han, and John Quiggin. 1997. "Characterizing QALYs under a General Rank Dependent Utility Model," *Journal of Risk and Uncertainty* (15): 151-165.

Brouwer, Roy, and Ian Bateman. 2005. "Benefits Transfer of Willingness to Pay Estimates and Functions for Health-risk Reductions: a Cross-country Study," *Journal of Health Economics* 24: 591-611.

Buzby, Jean, and Tanya Roberts. 1996. "ERS Updates U.S. Foodborne Disease Costs for Seven Pathogens," *Food Review* 19(3): 20-25.

Buzby, Jean, Tanya Roberts, C.T. Jordon Lin, and James MacDonald. 1996. *Bacterial Foodborne Disease: Medical Costs and Productivity Losses*, AER-741, USDA, Economic Research Service. Accessed April 2013 at: http://www.ers.usda.gov/publications/aer-agricultural-economic-report/aer741.aspx

Cameron, Trudy Ann, and J.R. DeShazo. 2013. "Demand for Health Risk Reductions," *Journal of Environmental Economics and Management* (65): 87-109.

Cropper, Maureen, Michael Greenstone, Michael Hanemann, Gloria Helfand, William Pizer, Lori Chestnut, James Hammitt, Reed Johnson, Kathleen Segerson, and V. Kerry Smith. 2007. *SAB Advisory on EPA's Issues in Valuing Mortality Risk Reduction*, EPA-SAB-08-001, Memorandum to U.S. Environmental Protection Agency Administrator Stephen L. Johnson from the EPA Science Advisory Board and Environmental Economics Advisory Committee. Accessed April 2013 at: http://nepis.epa.gov/Adobe/PDF/P10007U3.pdf

Crutchfield, Stephen, and Tanya Roberts. 2000. "Food Safety Efforts Accelerate in the 1990s,"*Food Review* (23): 44-49. Accessed April 2013 at: http://webarchives.cdlib.org/sw1bc3ts3z/http://ers.usda.gov/Publications/FoodReview/Septdec00/FRsept00h.pdf

Dickie, Mark, and John List. 2006. "Economic Valuation of Health for Environmental Policy: Comparing Alternative Approaches: Introduction and Overview," *Environmental and Resource Economics* (34): 339-46.

EuropQol Group. "About Us." Accessed March 25, 2013 at: http://www.euroqol.org/euroqol-group/about-us.html

Garg, Amit, Louise Moise, Douglas Matsell, Heather Thiessen-Philbrook, Brian Haynes, Rita Suri, Marina Salvadori, Joel Ray, and William Clark for the Walkerton Health Study Investigators. 2005. "Risk of Hypertension and Reduced Kidney Function after Acute Gastroenteritis from Bacteria-contaminated Drinking Water," *Canadian Medical Association Journal* 173(3): 261-68.

Gerking, Shelby, Mark Dickie, and Marcella Veronesi. 2012. *Valuation of Human Health: An Integrated Model of Willingness to Pay for Mortality and Morbidity Risk Reductions*, U.S. EPA, National Center for Environmental Economics, Working Paper 12-07, October 2012. Accessed April 2013 at: http://yosemite.epa.gov/ee/epa/eed.nsf/WPNumber/2012-07/$File/2012-07.pdf

Gold, Marthe, Joanna Siegel, Louise Russell, et al., eds. 1996. *Cost-Effectiveness in Health and Medicine*, New York, NY: Oxford University Press.

Gold, Marthe, David Stevenson, and Dennis Fryback. 2002. "QALYs and QALYs and DALYs, Oh My: Similarities and Differences in Summary Measures of Population Health," *Annual Review of Public Health* (23): 115-134.

Grosse, Scott, Steven Teutsch, and Anne Haddix. 2007. "Lessons on Cost Effectiveness in the US Public Health Policy," *Annual Review of Public Health* (28): 365-91.

Gyrd-Hansen, Dorte. 2003. "Willingness to Pay for a QALY," *Health Economics* 12(12): 1049-60.

Hammitt, James. 2008. "QALY vs. WTP," *Risk Analysis* 22(5): 985-1001.

Hammitt, James, and Kenneth Haninger. 2007. "Willingness to Pay for Food Safety: Sensitivity to Duration and Severity of Illness," *American Journal of Agricultural Economics* 89(5): 1170-75.

Hammitt, James, and Kenneth Haninger. 2010. "Valuing Fatal Risks to Children and Adults: Effects of Disease, Latency, and Risk Aversion," *Journal of Risk and Uncertainty* (40): 57-83.

Hammitt, James, and Kenneth Haninger. 2011. *Valuing Morbidity Risk: Willingness-to-pay per Quality-Adjusted Life Year,* Working Paper, March 2011. Accessed April 2013 at: http://neeo.univ-tlse1.fr/2877/1/11.09.343.pdf

Harberger, Arnold. (1971). "Three Basic Postulates for Applied Welfare Economics: An Interpretive Essay." *Journal of Economic Literature* 9(3): 785-797.

Harrington, Winston, and Paul Portney. 1987. "Valuing the Benefits of Health and Safety Regulation," *Journal of Urban Economics* 22(1): 101-12.

Hoffmann, Sandra, Michael Batz, and J. Glenn Morris Jr. 2012. "Annual Cost of Illness and Quality-Adjusted Life Year Losses in the United States Due to 14 Foodborne Pathogens," *Journal of Food Protection* 75(7): 1291-1302.

Hunt, Alistair, and Julia Ferguson. 2010. *A Review of Recent Policy-relevant Findings from the Environmental Health Literature*, Organisation for Economic Co-operation and Development, Environment Directorate, Environment Policy Committee. Feb. 16, 2010.

Institute of Medicine, National Academies of Science. 2006. *Valuing Health for Regulatory Cost-Effectiveness Analysis* (W. Miller, L.A. Robinson, and R.S. Lawrence, eds.). Washington, DC: National Academies Press.

Krupnick, Alan. 2007. "Mortality-risk Valuation and Age: Stated Preference Evidence," *Review of Environmental Economics and Policy* 1(2): 261-82.

Kuchler, Fred, and Elise Golan. 1999. *Assigning Values to Life: Comparing Methods for Valuing Health Risks*, AER-784, USDA, Economic Research Service.

Lipscomb, Michael, Dennis Fryback, Marthe Gold, and Dennis Revicki. 2009. "Retaining, and Enhancing, the QALY," *Value in Health* (12): s18-s26.

Lindhjem, Henrik, StäleNavrud, Nils Axel Braathen, and Vincent Biausque. 2011. "Valuing Mortality Risk Reductions from Environmental, Transport, and Health Policies: A Global Meta-Analysis of Stated Preference Studies," *Risk Analysis* 31(9): 1381-1407.

Marks, S., and Tanya Roberts. 1993. "*E. coli* O157:H7 Ranks as the Fourth Most Costly Foodborne Disease," *FoodReview* 16(3): 51-59.

Mead, Paul S., Laurence Slutsker, Vance Dietz, et al. 1999. "Food-related Illness and Death in the United States," *Emerging Infectious Diseases* (5): 607–25.

Minyamoto, J.M., P.P. Wakker, H. Bleichrodt, and H.J.M. Peters. 1998. "The Zero-Condition: A Simplifying Assumption in QALY Measurement and Multiattribute Utility," *Management Science* (44): 839-49.

Morris, J. Glenn, J. 2011. "How Safe is Our Food," *Emerging Infectious Diseases*. Accessed May 10, 2012 at: http://wwwnc.cdc.gov/eid/article/17/1/10-1821_article.htm

National Research Council. 2008. *Estimating Mortality Risk Reduction and Economic Benefits from Controlling Ozone Air Pollution*, Committee on Estimating Mortality Risk Reduction Benefits from Decreasing Tropospheric Ozone Exposure. Washington DC: National Academies Press.

Pliskin, J.S., D. Shepard, and Martin Weinstein. 1980. "Utility Functions for Life Years and Health Status," *Operations Research* (28): 206-24.

Pinot-Prades, Jose Luis, Graham Loomes, and Raul Brey. 2009. "Trying to Estimate a Monetary Value for the QALY," *Journal of Health Economics* (28):553-62.

Roberts, Tanya. 1989. "Human Illness Costs of Foodborne Bacteria," *American Journal of Agricultural Economics* 71(2): 468-74.

Roberts, Tanya, K.D. Murrell, and S. Marks. 1994. "Economic Losses Caused by Foodborne Parasitic Diseases," *Parasitology Today* 10(11): 419-23.

Robinson, Lisa, and James Hammitt. 2013. "Skills of the Trade: Valuing Health Risk Reductions in Benefit-Cost Analysis," *Journal of Benefit-Cost Analysis* 4(1): 107-130.

Scallan, Elaine, Robert M. Hoekstra, Frederick Angulo, et al. 2011a. "Foodborne Illness Acquired in the United States—Major Pathogens," *Emerging Infectious Diseases* (17): 7-15.

Scallan, Elaine, Patricia Griffin, Frederick Angulo, et al. 2011b. "Foodborne Illness Acquired in the United States–Unspecified Agents," *Emerging Infectious Diseases* (17): 16-22.

Scharff, Robert. 2010. *Health-related Costs from Foodborne Illness in the United States.* Produce Safety Project, Georgetown University. Accessed January 2013 at http://www.marlerblog.com/ uploads/image/PSP-Scharff%20v9.pdf

Scharff, Robert. 2012. "Economic Burden from Health Losses Due to Foodborne Illness in the United States," *Journal of Food Protection* 75(1): 123-31.

Shaw, J. W., J. A. Johnson, and S. J. Coons. 2005. "U.S. Valuation of the EQ-5D Health States: Development and Testing of the D1 Valuation Model," *Medical Care* (43): 203-30.

Shepard, Donald, and Richard Zeckhauser. 1984. "Survival versus Consumption," *Management Science* (30): 423-39.

Slovic, Paul. 1987. "Perception of Risk," *Science* 236(4799): 280-85.

Steahr, T., and Tanya Roberts. 1993. *Microbial Foodborne Disease: Hospitalizations, Medical Costs and Potential Demand for Safer Food*, Working Paper WP-32, presented at Private Strategies, Public Policies, and Food System Performance conference.

Tolley, George, Donald Kenkel, and Robert Fabian (eds.). 1994. *Valuing Health for Policy: An Economic Approach*, Chicago, IL: University of Chicago Press.

U.S. Centers for Disease Control and Prevention (CDC). *FastStats: Health Expenditures.* Accessed March 2013 at http://www.cdc.gov/nchs/fastats/hexpense.htm

U.S. Congress. Aug. 3, 1993. *Government Performance Results Act of 1993*, Public Law 103-62. Accessed at http://www.whitehouse.gov/omb/mgmt-gpra/gplaw2m, on May 10, 2012. As amended by U.S. Congress (Jan. 4, 2011) *Government Performance, Results and Accountability Modernization Act of 2010*, Public Law 111-352. Accessed May 2012 at http://www.gpo.gov/ fdsys/pkg/BILLS-111hr2142enr/pdf/BILLS-111hr2142enr.pdf

U.S. Congress. Jan. 4, 2011. *Food Safety Modernization Act of 2010*, Public Law 111-353. Accessed at http://www.gpo.gov/fdsys/pkg/PLAW-111publ353/pdf/PLAW-111publ353.pdf

U.S. Department of Agriculture, Economic Research Service. *Food Expenditures.* Accessed March 2013 at http://www.ers.usda.gov/data-products/food-expenditures.aspx

U.S. Department of Agriculture, Economic Research Service. Foodborne Illness Cost Calculator. Accessed April 2012 at http://webarchives.cdlib.org/sw1rf5mh0k/http:/www.ers.usda.gov/Data/ FoodborneIllness/

U.S. Environmental Protection Agency. 2010a. *Guidelines for Preparing Economic Analysis.* Accessed May 2012 at http://yosemite.epa.gov/ee/epa/eerm.nsf/vwAN/EE-0568-52.pdf/$file/ EE-0568-52.pdf

U.S. Environmental Protection Agency. 2010b. *Valuing Mortality Risk Reductions for Environmental Protection: A White Paper, SAB Review Draft.* Dec. 10, 2010. Accessed February 2013 at http://yosemite.epa.gov/ee/epa/eerm.nsf/vwAN/EE-0563-1.pdf/$file/EE-0563-1.pdf

U.S. Food and Drug Administration. 2012. *Bad Bug Book, 2nd Edition: Foodborne Pathogenic Microorganisms and Natural Toxins Handbook*. Accessed May 2012 at http://www.fda.gov/food/foodsafety/foodborneillness/foodborneillnessfoodbornepathogensnaturaltoxins/badbugbook/default.htm

U.S. Office of Management and Budget. Sept. 17, 2003. *Circular A-4. Regulatory Analysis*. Accessed May 2012 at http://www.whitehouse.gov/sites/default/files/omb/assets/omb/circulars/a004/a-4.pdf

Vassanadumrongdee, Sujitra, Shunji Matsuoka, and Hiroaki Shirakawa. 2004. "Meta-analysis of Contingent Valuation Studies on Air Pollution-related Morbidity Risks," *Environmental Economics and Policy Studies* (6): 11-47.

Viscusi, W. Kip. 2008. "How to Value a Life," *Journal of Economics and Finance* (28): 311-23.

Viscusi, W. Kip, and Joseph Aldy. 2003. "The Value of a Statistical Life: A Critical Review of Market Estimates Throughout the World," *Journal of Risk and Uncertainty* (27): 5-76.

Viscusi, W. Kip, Joel Huber, and Jason Bell. 2012. "Heterogeneity in Values of Morbidity Risks from Drinking Water," *Environmental and Resource Economics* (52): 23-48.

Zeckhauser, Richard, and Donald Shepard. 1976. "Where Now for Saving Lives?" *Law and Contemporary Problems* 40(4): 5-45.

Appendix

There is broad consensus that cost-of-illness measures usually underestimate the public's willingness to pay for programs that reduce the risk of nonfatal illness (Viscusi, 2008). But cost-of-illness estimates continue to be used because there are often no readily available, low-cost alternatives. This has been a major motivating factor behind the practice of including monetized QALY estimates in monetary estimates of the burden of illness. Analyzing the benefits of programs that reduce the risk of nonfatal illness would be much more tractable if one could simply monetize a nondisease-specific QALY metric, like those based on the EQ-5D. But realizing this vision raises a number of theoretical and empirical questions.

A fundamental theoretical question is whether QALY loss represents preferences in the way these are defined in economics. If not, then the meaning of such estimates would be unclear. QALY loss is defined as a constant health-quality weight for a health state times duration of that health state. This implies that individuals' preferences over health states are independent of their preferences over how long they spend in the health state, the age at which the state is experienced, and the individual's remaining life expectancy (Pliskin et al., 1980), or, alternatively, that individuals are risk-neutral over longevity given quality of life (Bleichrodt et al., 1997; Miyamoto et al., 1998).[5] While empirical research shows that these conditions are often not met, there is debate over whether these empirical violations are large enough to invalidate interpretation of QALYs as a proper utility function in the context of standard economic theory (Hammitt, 2008, Robinson and Hammitt (2013).

In policy analysis, current practice is to value QALY loss by multiplying it by the VSLY, building on work by Tolley et al. (1994) (IoM, 2006). The VSLY is assumed to be constant and calculated as the average VSL for a population divided by average remaining life expectancy of that population discounted to present value (Robinson and Hammitt (2003). In a simplified example taken from Robinson and Hammitt (2013), if there were no discounting and the average age of a population in a study that estimates a VSL of $6 million is 40 with an average life expectancy of 75, then the VSLY would be $6 million divided by 35 or $279,000.[6] Being constant means that the VSLY does not vary with gains in life expectancy which, in turn, implies that the VSL is proportional to remaining life expectancy.

The practice of using a constant VSLY to value QALYs has been the focus of much of the recent research literature on valuation of QALYs. Theoretically, if capital markets were perfect and individuals could borrow over their entire lifespan, then the VSLY could be constant over the course of a life (Rosen, 1988). If, as is more typical, the ability to borrow against future income is limited, the VSL and VSLY likely will rise and then fall, peaking in middle age (Shepard and Zeckhauser, 1984). Aldy and Viscusi (2007) provide a clear, nonmathematical review of this literature. There is a sizeable empirical literature on how the VSL changes with factors correlated with life expectancy—age, gender, and income. Recent reviews of these studies find some evidence that the VSL varies with age (Krupnick et al., 2007; Aldy and Viscusi, 2007). A recent review of labor market studies

---

[5]Risk neutrality over longevity means that individuals are indifferent between gambles over different possible longevity with different probabilities as long as all the gambles have the same expected longevity. For example, risk neutrality over longevity implies that a 50-year-old would be indifferent between a medical treatment option that carried a 50-percent probability of living to 85 but also a 50-percent probability of only living to 55 and a medical option that carried a 100-percent probability of living to 70.

[6]The ERS Foodborne Illness Cost Calculator, developed in the early 2000s, provided a more sophisticated explanation, interpreting the VSL as the present discounted value of a stream of constant annuity payments over the remaining lifetime of an average 40-year-old man.

finds that the VSL and VSLY rise until middle age and then decline over the rest of life, and that, contrary to Rosen's (1998) theoretical model, the VSL is lower at 20 years old than at 60 years old, despite obvious differences in life expectancy (Aldy and Viscusi, 2007).

Beyond debate about use of a *constant* VSLY to monetize QALYs, there lies the question of whether it is even appropriate to use the VSL (WTP to reduce small risks of *death*) as a proxy for WTP to reduce risk of nonfatal *illness*. OMB guidance advises agencies using secondary research as a source of valuation estimates to choose studies in which the good and magnitude of the good being valued are similar to that expected to be provided by the regulation (OMB, 2003). VSL estimates currently used in regulatory analysis are based primarily on studies of WTP to reduce risk of fatal workplace or automobile accidents (U.S. EPA, 2010a; U.S. EPA, 2010b). It is unclear how these studies, involving deaths that are generally not preceded by extended morbidity, relate to WTP to reduce the risk of nonfatal illnesses like moderate diarrhea or chronic irritable bowel syndrome. There is some evidence that the VSL varies by cause of death, which in turn could be related to preferences over morbidity (Adamowicz et al., 2011). For example, some studies find a "premium" for reducing risk of death from cancer compared to death from accidents (EPA, 2010b). But EPA's Scientific Advisory Board does not feel that these findings are strong enough to support use of a "cancer premium" in EPA regulatory analysis, and it is unclear whether preferences over predeath morbidity or attitudes like dread of cancer drive any "premium" that does exist (EPA, 2010b). New research looking at WTP for reduction in the risk of death preceded by a period of morbidity will give insight into the relationship between WTP to reduce risk of death and risk of illness and what this might mean for VSLY estimates (Cameron and DeShazo, 2013; Gerking et al., 2012).